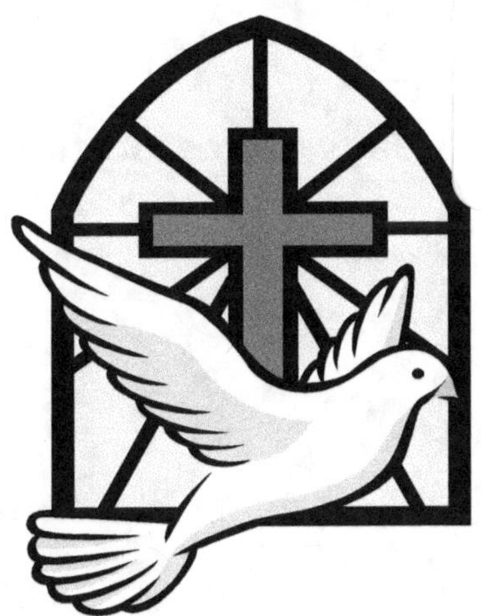

30 Days of Restoration

Shed your Flesh to Gain in your Spirit

BY T'aira Lynn Jones

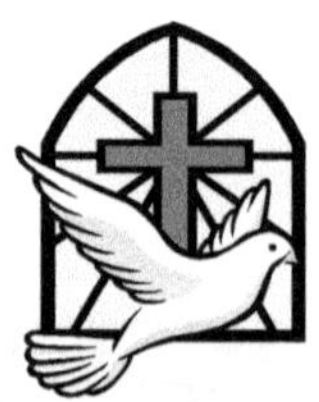

30 Days of Restoration

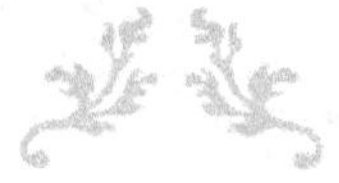

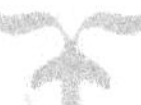

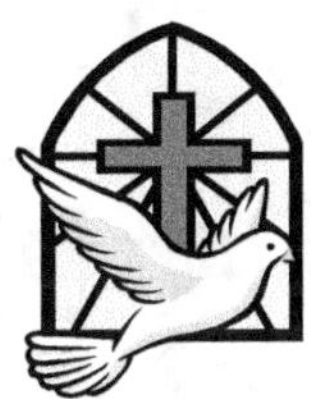 **30 Days of Restoration**

Introduction

Our bodies are made up into three parts; body, soul, and spirit. The body is considered your flesh. The part you can touch, feel, taste, hear, and see. However, the body is just a puppet that it is subject to the other soul and spirit. The soul is what contains your personality. It determines our emotions, our feelings, our desires, our wants, and our intellect. The soul only falls subject to the spirit. The spirit is where Jesus rests. (As long as we are born again). Therefore, if God doesn't dwell in you, then you are in darkness, and you can't control the soul and body.

> *1 John 2:11 "But he that hateth his brother is in darkness, and walketh in darkness, and knoweth not whither he goeth, because that darkness hath blinded his eyes."*

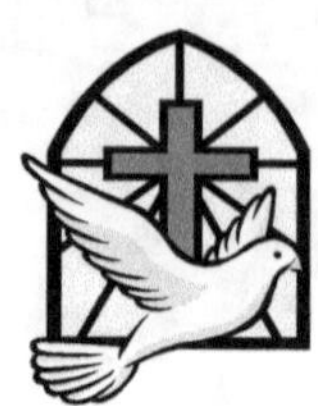 # 30 Days of Restoration

This 30-day plan is not just another weight-loss tactic. Rather, it is a beginning of a clean life working from the inside to the outside. If you think that doing this half way or not sticking to the whole plan is going to benefit you—it won't. If you believe that it is going to be some overnight miracle—it won't. On the other hand, if you **are** determined to change and become a healthier you, so that God can use you with out the side effects, then this will the beginning to a new way of living. It will be one of the best changes that you will do, because you are doing this by putting God first.

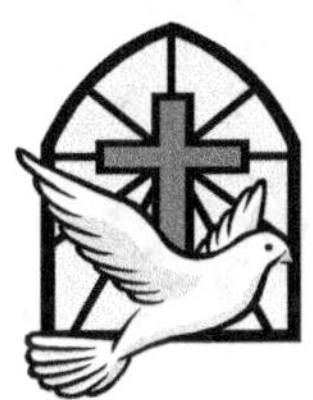

30 Days of Restoration

PREFACE

Now how exactly will this restoration benefit you?

> *Isaiah 40:31 "But they that wait upon the Lord shall renew their strength; they shall mount up with wings as eagles; they shall run, and not be weary; and they shall walk, and not faint."*

Think of an eagle. It is the most majestic and strongest bird alive. When people speak of this bird they think freedom, life, and strength. Eagles must go through a restoration process to grow from a babe to an adult. The eagle must go through a grueling shedding process which consist of plucking its feathers, bashing its beak on the ground until the old beak comes off, and pulling its talons. During that five-month period the eagle has to seclude itself from everything that may bring it harm or even death. As its beak, feathers, and talons regenerate they return stronger and thicker. While the restoration process may seem painful at first, it is beneficial and needful for the eagle to survive and live longer. So just like the eagle, we also must shed some things off us. Things that are not beneficial to our bodies, like empty calories.

Consider what you want God to do in your life during this 30-day plan. You want God to do something amazing right? Beyond your imagination? What sacrifice of thanks are you giving Him? Do you turn down your plate, or turn off the television an hour earlier? Or just stop in the middle of your crazy busy day to think on Him, pray, or study the word. The Lord really desires more from you.

Do not get content in your way of life just because you have lived a certain way all these years. Because contentment always brings and puts on extra baggage, which can cloud your judgment. Think of couch potatoes. If all they did was sit, eat, and watch TV all day they are going to become obese. If you take a bin and fill it up with trash you are going to get a garbage bin. If you take that same bin and fill it up with flowers, it changes from a garbage bin to a flower bin. So, when you sit on the couch all day eating with

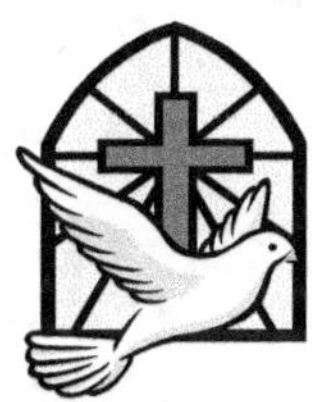

your eyes and ears the things of this world; you become worldly. So, do as the word of God tells you.

> **Romans 12:2 KJV And be not conformed to this world: but be ye transformed by the renewing of your mind, that ye may prove what is that good, and acceptable, and perfect, will of God.**

Challenge yourself to do better in Jesus. Study the bible a little longer, pray a little harder, and seek Him daily. You need to strive for perfection in your relationship with Christ.

> **Hebrews 11:6 "But without faith it is impossible to please Him: for that cometh to God must believe that He is, and that He is a rewarder of them that diligently seek Him."**

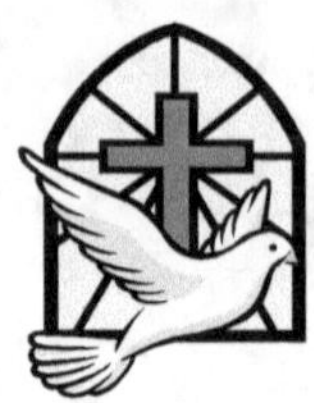

30 Days of Restoration

Dear Heavenly Father,

I want to thank you for keeping my life thus far. I know that you have a plan for my life and everything is ordained by you. I will no longer accept the fact that I can't change because all things are possible in you. Jesus, I am asking for Your power to overcome this flesh. I am going to dedicate the next thirty days to You and Your will. I am going to make healthier choices for my life. Help my spirit to become strengthened and empowered so that I might be able to stand and resist the enemy. I praise you and thank you in advance for everything that you are going to do in the days to come. In Jesus name I pray.....Amen.

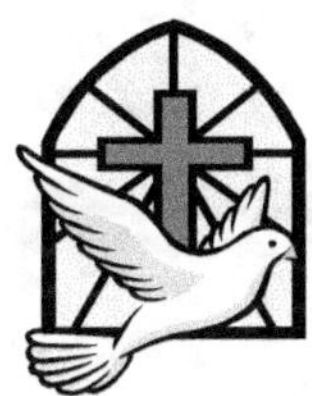

30 Days of Restoration

Week 1

This week your body will go through both physical and emotional changes. Your soul is going to crave something and your body will react to that craving by trying to grab it. However, you are going to have to use your spirit to control your soul and body. This will be the hardest week of all, but do not be discouraged. You are more than capable of making it through. You have made the biggest leap of faith by first identifying that you need restoration. The main resource to overcome this week is prayer.

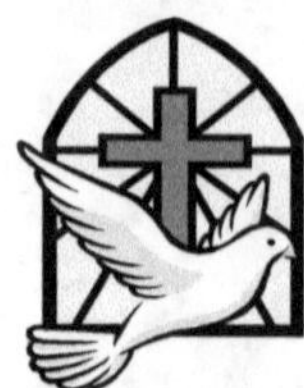

30 Days of Restoration

Matthew 21:22 "And all things, whatsoever ye shall seek in prayer, believing, you shall receive. So, pray and believe that this week you will conquer your flesh."

Foods for restoration:

Fruit *(raw-cooked-steamed)*
Vegetables *(raw-cooked-steamed)*
Potato *(whole with skin)*
Rice *(preferably brown or wild)*
Beans *(lentils, black eyed peas, red, etc)*
Water (unsweetened tea)
Spices: *olive oil, vinegar, pepper, any Herbs, may use sugar substitute sparingly*

Foods on restriction:

Meat
Bread/pasta
Sugar
Salt
Dairy
Butter

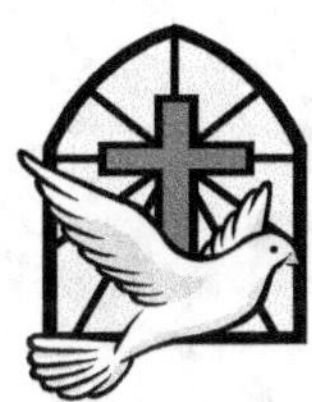

30 Days of Restoration

Be inventive and creative with your meals. You can have as much as you want of the restorative foods, there is no limit on amounts. However, keep in mind that you are making a lifestyle change, so you do not want to overdo it. You should eat only the amount that is needed for your body. So, if work in an office or sit down most of the day then you should eat less of the rice or potatoes and eat more of the beans and vegetables. And vice versa if you are more active at work; but still, keep a healthy balance. Note: Your bowel movements will become more regular. Make sure you are drinking plenty of water during this time.

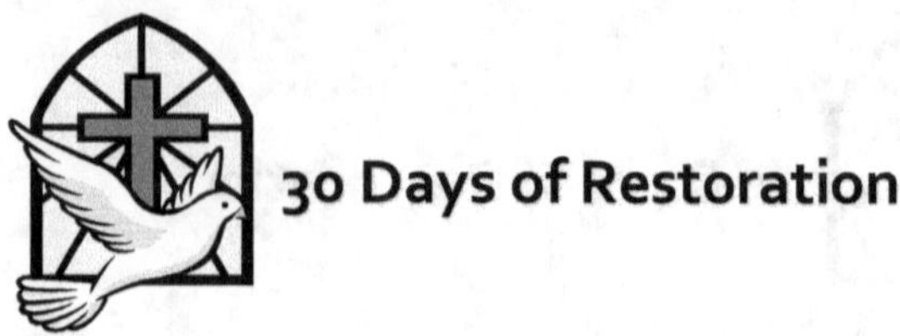

Daily Scriptures

Days 1-7

<u>Day 1</u>

Deuteronomy 30:19

I call heaven and earth to record this day against you, that I have set before you life and death, blessing and cursing: therefore choose life, that both thou and thy seed may live: 20 That thou mayest love the LORD thy God, and that thou mayest obey his voice, and that thou mayest cleave unto him: for he is thy life, and the length of thy days: that thou mayest dwell in the land which the LORD sware unto thy fathers, to Abraham, to Isaac, and to Jacob, to give them.

Day 2

Proverbs 14:26

In the fear of the LORD is strong confidence: and his children shall have a place of refuge.

Day 3

2 Samuel 22:30

For by thee I have run through a troop: by my God have I leaped over a wall.

Day 4

Philippians 3:13

Brethren, I count not myself to have apprehended: but this one thing I do, forgetting those things which are behind, and reaching forth unto those things which are before.

Day 5

Romans 6:17

But God be thanked, that ye were the servants of sin, but ye have obeyed from the heart that form of doctrine which was delivered you.

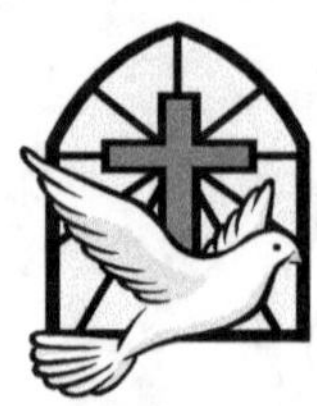

30 Days of Restoration

Day 6

1Corinthians 9:27

But I keep under my body, and bring it into subjection: lest that by any means, when I have preached to others, I myself should be a castaway.

Day 7

1Corinthians 10:13

There hath no temptation taken you but such as is common to man: but God is faithful, who will not suffer you to be tempted above that ye are able; but will with the temptation also make a way to escape, that ye may be able to bear it.

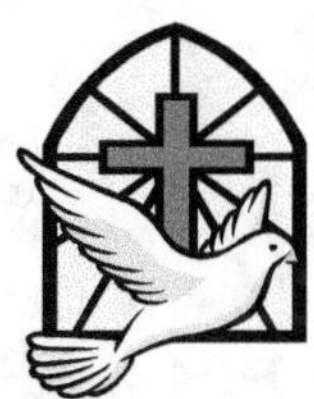

30 Days of Restoration

Notes

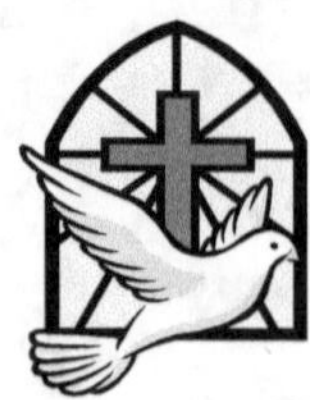 **30 Days of Restoration**

Now give God the praise, honor, and the glory, because you have made it through the first week. At this point your body has been through a physical wake up call. You are starting to breakdown harmful toxins that you have put in your body over many years. Your soul has gone through emotional strain because you have denied it what it desires. All in all, your spirit is strengthening because you have learned to shed your flesh.

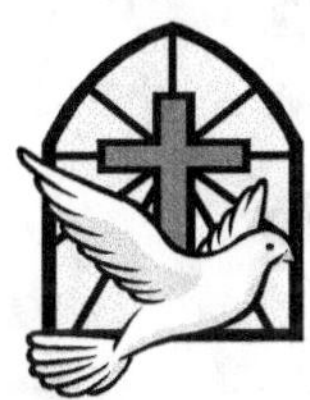

30 Days of Restoration

Foods for restoration:

Vegetables-raw-cooked-steamed

Potato (whole with skin)

Rice (preferably brown or wild)

Beans (lentils, black eyed peas, red, etc)

Add one meat a day-Chicken, Turkey, or fish only

Add 2 serving of dairy-milk (preferably almond, rice, or soy), cheese, nonfat yogurt

*Water-unsweetened tea-*100% fruit juice*

Spices: olive oil, vinegar, pepper, any Herbs may use sugar substitute sparingly

Foods to restriction:

Bread/Pasta

Sugar

Salt

Fruit

Butter

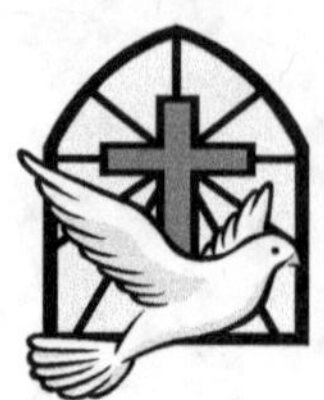

Don't think to yourself that you can't make it, or this is a bad thing. But cast the enemy out of your mind because right now the Lord is being glorified in you, through your sacrifice.

You can now have meat this week; but only once a day. And YES, eggs are considered meat. Pick and choose you meals wisely. Do not fry and batter your chicken. Come up with your own different recipes to cook your meat.

Try something like Chicken stuffed with tomatoes and mozzarella cheese. Read the labels to find out the true serving sizes are and stick to them.

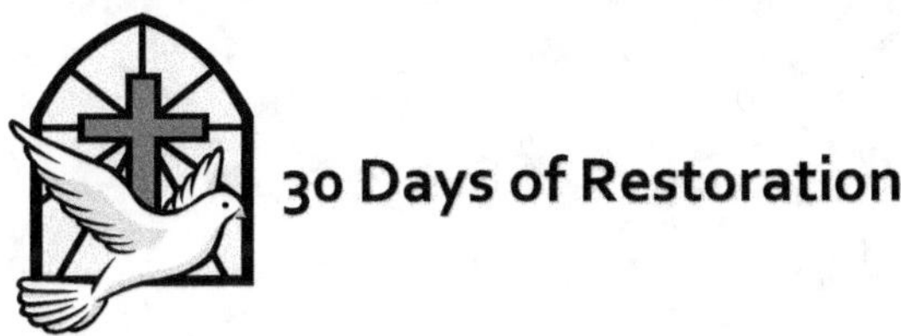

30 Days of Restoration

Daily Scripture

Day 8-14

DAY 8

Galatians 6:9

And let us not be weary in well doing: for in due season we shall reap, if we faint not

DAY 9

Proverbs 21:21

He that followeth after righteousness and mercy findeth life, righteousness, and honour.

DAY 10

Psalm 90:12

So teach us to number our days, that we may apply our hearts unto wisdom.

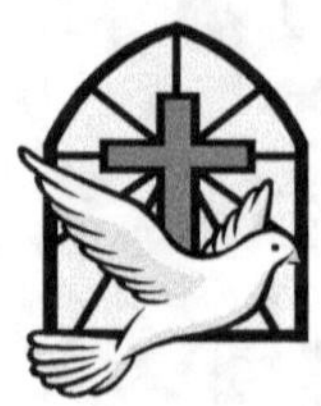

30 Days of Restoration

DAY 11
1 Corinthians 6:12
All things are lawful unto me, but all things are not expedient: all things are lawful for me, but I will not be brought under the power of any.

Day 12
Romans 12:2
And be not conformed to this world: but be ye transformed by the renewing of your mind, that ye may prove what is that good, and acceptable, and perfect, will of God.

DAY 13
1 Peter 3:10
For he that will love life, and see good days, let him refrain his tongue from evil, and his lips that they speak no guile:

DAY 14
Isaiah 26:3
Thou wilt keep him in perfect peace, whose mind is stayed on thee: because he trusteth in thee.

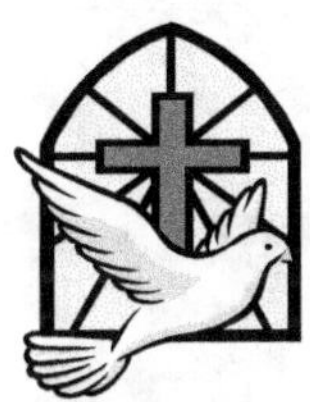

30 Days of Restoration

**Notes

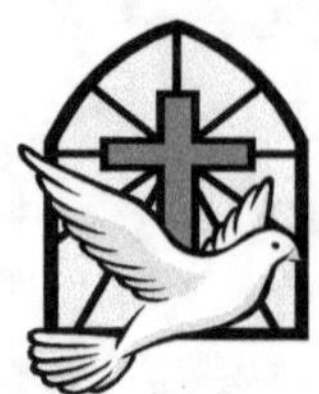

30 Days of Restoration

Week 3

Jesus has blessed and kept you. You are not dead but yet alive. You are now half way through this plan. Glory be to God. Keep in mind that you are using this time to shed your flesh while at the same time working on your relationship with God.

> ***Mathew 5:6 Blessed are they which do hunger and thirst after righteousness: for they shall be filled.***

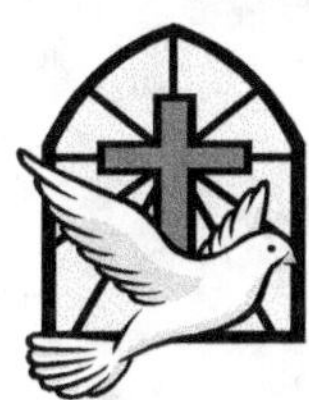 # 30 Days of Restoration

So, give Him more of your time to pray and read His word. Fatten your spirit by gaining knowledge of His word and asking Him about what He wants from you. Spend time with your family and your church family. Set aside time to spend some quality time with your family, friends, or church group. This should be true bonding time with one another without argument or strife. Try without distractions!

<u>Foods for restoration:</u>

Fruit (raw-cooked)
Vegetables-(raw-cooked-steamed
Potato (whole with skin)
Rice (preferably brown or wild)
Beans (lentils, black eyed peas, red, etc)
***2 serving of meats a day-Chicken, Turkey, or fish only**
***2 serving of dairy-milk, cheese, nonfat yogurt**
Water-unsweetened tea-*100% fruit juice
Spices: olive oil, vinegar, pepper, any Herbs may use sugar substitute sparingly

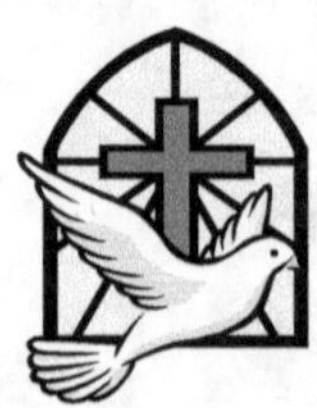

30 Days of Restoration

<u>Foods for restriction:</u>
Bread/Pasta
Sugar
Salt
Butter

Your energy should be through the roof. So use it. Get out and walk. Start out walking for just ten minutes and increase time by five minutes each day. If you sit at work all day, move your feet and burn some energy. Set your chair setting on the lowest bar which will cause you to use more energy to get in and out of it.

Try little things like parking further away from your job or the store. Get physically motivated. Pick up some small weights and do arms curls while reading. Be your own physical trainer by pushing yourself pass your limits, so you can do better and achieve more.

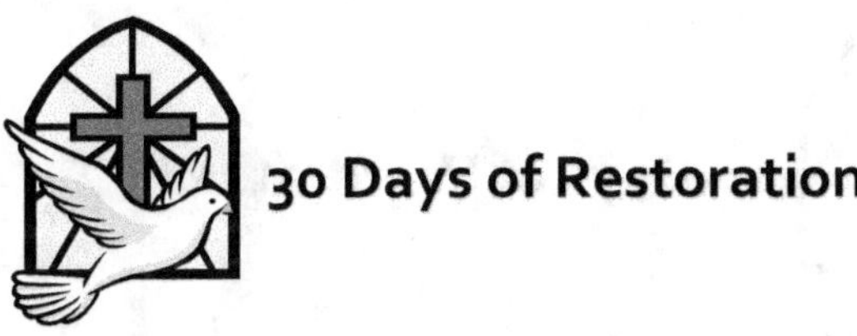

Daily Scripture

Day 15-21

DAY 15

Psalm 5:3

My voice shalt thou hear in the morning, O LORD; in the morning will I direct my prayer unto thee, and will look up.

DAY 16

Psalm 103:2-5

Bless the LORD, O my soul, and forget not all his benefits:Who forgiveth all thine iniquities; who healeth all thy diseases; Who redeemeth thy life from destruction; who crowneth thee with lovingkindness and tender mercies; Who satisfieth thy mouth with good things; so that thy youth is renewed like the eagle's.

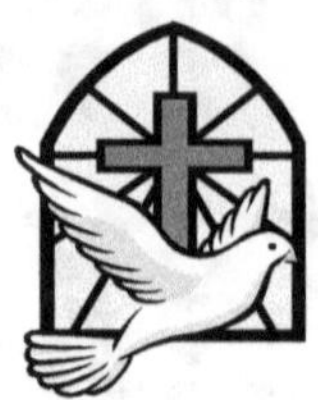

30 Days of Restoration

DAY 17
Proverbs 31:27
She looketh well to the ways of her household, and eateth not the bread of idleness.

DAY 18
Ecclesiastes 4:9, 12
Two are better than one; because they have a good reward for their labour. And if one prevail against him, two shall withstand him; and a threefold cord is not quickly broken.

DAY 19
Proverbs 25:28
He that hath no rule over his own spirit is like a city that is broken down, and without walls.

DAY 20
Luke 16:10
He that is faithful in that which is least is faithful also in much: and he that is unjust in the least is unjust also in much.

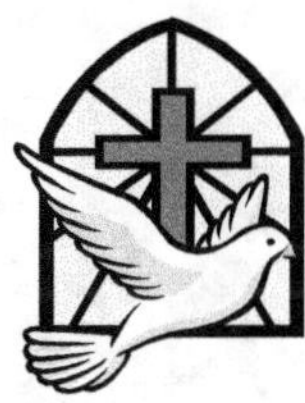

30 Days of Restoration

DAY 21
Psalm 141:3-4
Set a watch, O LORD, before my mouth; keep the door of my lips. Incline not my heart to any evil thing, to practice wicked works with men that work iniquity: and let me not eat of their dainties.

Notes

Week 4

Do you feel that wind? Because you have just breezed through this plan. You have gone through physical and mental changes. You should be able to breathe a little better because this is the last week. Think about the progress you have made thus far. God has blessed you with the power to overcome your worst enemy, yourself. Your spirit is much stronger because you have trusted in Jesus.

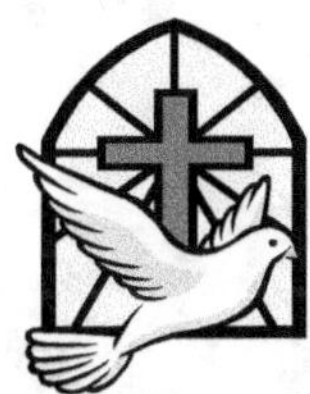

30 Days of Restoration

Foods for restoration:

Fruit (raw-cooked)

Vegetables (raw-cooked-steamed)

Potato (whole with skin)

Rice (preferably brown or wild)

Beans (lentils, black eyed peas, red, etc)

2 serving of meats a day-Chicken, Turkey, pork or fish only

2 serving of dairy-milk, cheese, nonfat yogurt

Add some salt and butter gradually

*Water-unsweetened tea-*100% fruit juice*

Spices: olive oil, vinegar, pepper, any Herbs may use sugar substitute sparingly

Foods for restricting:

Bread/Pasta

Sugar

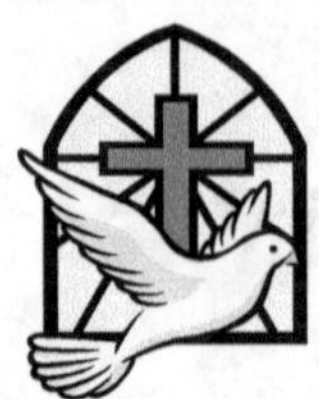

30 Days of Restoration

Look back to week one and remember where you started. You might have had thoughts of defeat and opposition to beginning this lifestyle change. But look at you now!

Every cell in your body is celebrating your new life because it is not clouded by toxins. Your blood pressure should be better. Your glucose level should be lowered. Overall you are completely different because your mindset has changed.

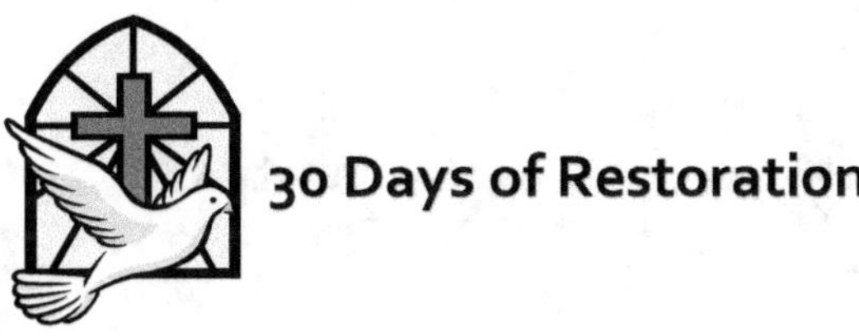

30 Days of Restoration

Daily Scriptures

Day 22-28

Day 22

Proverbs 25:27

It is not good to eat much honey: so for men to search their own glory is not glory.

Day23

Hebrews 6:11-12

And we desire that every one of you do shew the same diligence to the full assurance of hope unto the end: That ye be not slothful, but followers of them who through faith and patience inherit the promises.

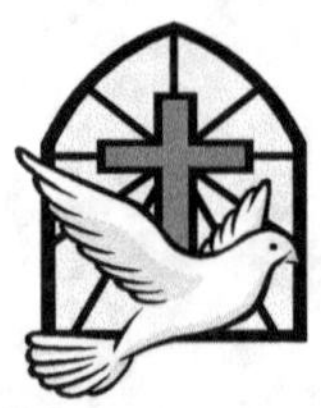

30 Days of Restoration

Day 24
Psalm 90:14

O satisfy us early with thy mercy; that we may rejoice and be glad all our days.

Day25
Isaiah 43:10

Ye are my witnesses, saith the LORD, and my servant whom I have chosen: that ye may know and believe me, and understand that I am he: before me there was no God formed, neither shall there be after me.

Day 26
Galatians 5:16

This I say then, Walk in the Spirit, and ye shall not fulfil the lust of the flesh.

Day 27
2 Corinthians 2:14

Now thanks be unto God, which always causeth us to triumph in Christ, and maketh manifest the savour of his knowledge by us in every place.

30 Days of Restoration

<u>Day28</u>
Isaiah 41:10

Fear thou not; for I am with thee: be not dismayed; for I am thy God: I will strengthen thee; yea, I will help thee; yea, I will uphold thee with the right hand of my righteousness.

Notes

____

____

____

____

____

____

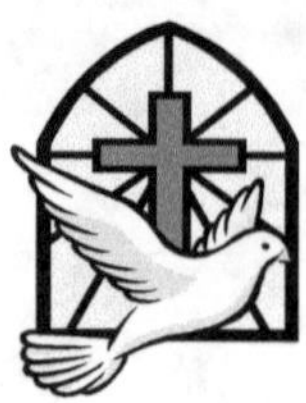

Week 5 and beyond

Day 29, 30 and beyond!

Praise Jehovah. You have made it through the end. You stayed strong and endured to the finish. Look at all the progress you have made from the beginning until now. Your body is now completely rid of all toxins. You are cleansed inside and out. Now where do we go from here? Make the right choices. God has given us the will to make choices for ourselves. He has provided the tools and resources to help us make the right ones.

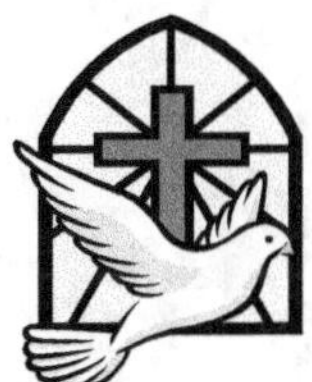

30 Days of Restoration

> *Philippians 4:13 I press toward the mark for the prize of the high calling of God in Christ Jesus.*

So make a stand for yourself to continue to be a healthier you. Do not go back to the old ways but move forward.

> *Philippians 3:13 Brethren, I count not myself to have apprehended; but this one thing I do, forgetting those things which are behind, and reaching forth unto those things which are before.*

Your new life has begun. Put God first so that you may be healthy in your body, soul and spirit.

<u>**Foods for restoration:**</u>

Gradually add to your diet if you so desire:

Sweets

Fats

Bread

Beef

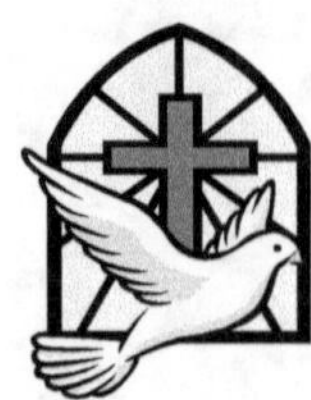

30 Days of Restoration

<u>Foods to restriction:</u>

Note:

Having made it this far without them. Please don't add these items all at once or you will become sick because your body will not be able to handle them anymore. If you do the little, God will always make it great.

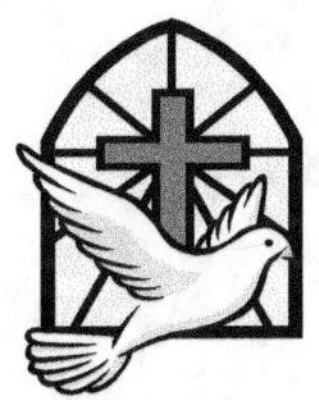

Closing Prayer

Dear Heavenly Father,

Thank you for this time of peace and restoration. I thank you for this experience that has brought restorative healing to my body. From this day forward, I promise to put you first and keep your first in my life. Lord, I will consult you with things concerning every aspect of my body, soul, and sprit. Continue to bless me with strength and endurance to continue to conquer my flesh in order to gain in my spirit.

In Jesus' name

Amen.

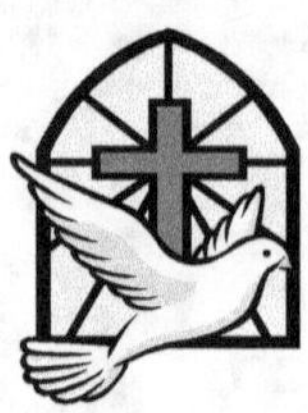

30 Days of Restoration

Notes

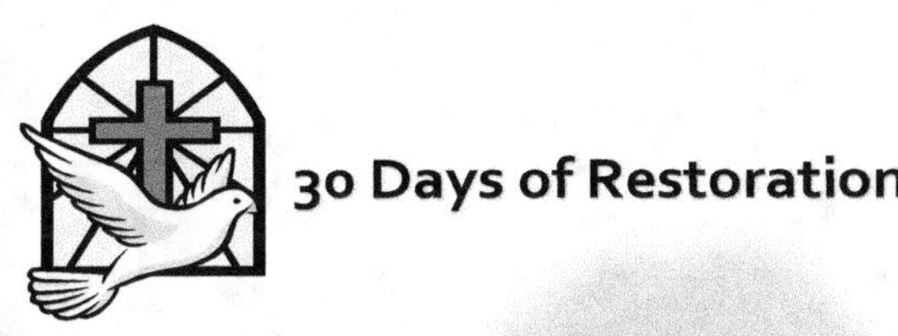

30 Days of Restoration

Special Thanks!

First, to my Lord and Savior Jesus Christ. To my loving and supportive husband Maurice. To my beautiful daughters Kennedy and Micah. A special thanks to my sister Ta'lor. For the support of all my friends and family. Finally, to my church family that gave me the inspiration to write this book.

May the Lord bless thee and keep thee!

Amen!